KETOGI
DIET

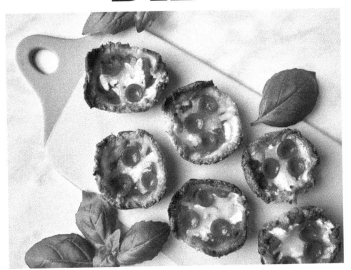

SNACKS
COOKBOOK

Felicity Flinn

Table of Contents

SNACKS

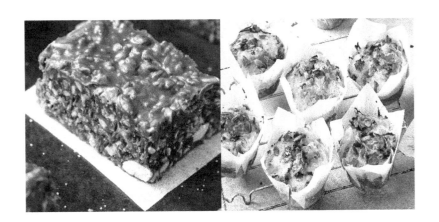

Graham Crackers Homemade

(Ready in about 20 mins| serving 10 | Difficulty: easy)

Per serving: kcal 156, Fat: 13.3g, net carbs:6.2g, Protein:5.21g

Ingredients

- Almond flour 2 cups
- Swerve brown 1/3 cup
- Cinnamon es2 tsp
- Baking powder 1 tsp
- Pinch salt
- Large egg 1
- Butter melted 2 tbsp
- Vanilla extract 1 tsp

Instructions

1. The oven preheated to 300f for crackers.

2. Whisk the almond/coconut flour, sweetener, spice, baking powder/soda & salt together in a big dish. Add the sugar, softened butter, black treacle & vanilla extract before the dough is combined.

3. Place the dough onto a wide sheet of bakery release paper or filler it with silicone, then pat it into a harsh rectangle. Cover it with such A single sheet of paper. Roll the dough as thinly if possible, To a thickness of around 1/8-1/4 inches.

4. Take Off The top parchment & use the knife or even a pizza Cutter to grade approximately 2 × 2 inches into squares. Place the whole parchment on a cookie sheet.

5. Bake for 20-30 mins, till it becomes brown & strong. Remove crackers, let them cool for 30 Mins, then break down together with score points. Go to a warm oven. Let mix it for the other 30 mins then allow It to cool fully (they crisp up while they cool).

Keto Cinnamon Roll Biscotti

(Ready in about 1hour 20 mins| serving 15 biscotti | Difficulty: medium)

Per serving: kcal 133, Fat: 12g, Net carbs:4g, Protein:5.21g

Ingredients

Filling/topping:

- Swerve sweetener 2 tbsp
- Ground cinnamon 1 tsp

Biscotti:

- Almond flour Honeyville 2 cups
- Swerve sweetener 1/3 cup
- Baking powder 1 tsp
- Xanthan gum 1/2 tsp
- Salt 1/4 tsp

- Melted butter+1 tbsp brushing biscotti 1/4 cup

- Large egg 1

- Vanilla extract 1 tsp

Glaze:

- Powdered Swerve sweetener 1/4 cup

- Heavy cream 2 tbsp

- Vanilla 1/2 tsp

Instructions

1. Mix sweetener & spice into A tiny bowl for filling. Place On aside.

2. Oven preheated to 325f, & line A bakery release paper baking sheet.

3. Whisk the almond/coconut flour, sweetener, baking soda/powder, Xanthan gum & salt together in the bowl. Mix the flour, egg & vanilla 1/4 Cup extract before the dough gets around.

4. Turn the dough on a cookie sheet and split it in two. The form could half into the ten by a four-inch rectangle. Ensure the size & form of both parts are comparable.

5. Sprinkle around 2/3 of cinnamon filling in one part. Place its other half of the dough on top and close that seams & smooth the surface.

6. Bake for 25 mins or until mildly Browned, then only tap solid. Remove the remaining melted butter from the oven and sweep, then dust it with the remaining cinnamon combination. Let it cool for 30 mins, And-the oven to cool down to 250f.

7. Slice logs into around 15 pieces using the fine knife

8. Put slices back on a cookie sheet and bake it for 15 Min, then turn over and bake it for another 15 min. Turn the oven off & Let stay away until it's cold.

9. For the glaze, mix powdered sweetener along with vanilla & cream extract until smooth. Drizzle on Chilled biscotti.

Strawberry Cheesecake Popsicles – Low-Carb and Gluten-Free

(Ready in about 4hour 15 mins| serving 12 popsicles | Difficulty: hard)

Per serving: kcal 122, Fat: 12g, Net carbs:3g, Protein:2g

Ingredients

- Softened cream cheese 8 oz
- Cream 1 cup
- Powdered Swerve sweetener 1/3 cup
- Stevia extract 1/4 tsp
- Lemon juice 1 tbsp
- Lemon zest 2 tsp
- Chopped fresh strawberries 2 cups

Instructions

1. Place and heat your "cream-cheese" In the mixing bowl until smooth.
2. Add milk powder swerve, lime Juice, stevia extract & lemon zest. Mixed phase till well.
3. Attach 1 1/2 cups of raspberries & finish processing until completely smooth. Delete Sliced leftover raspberries.
4. Pour the mixture into molds of popsicle & push Sticks of popsicle around two/three of the way in each.
5. Freeze it for 4 hrs. Run for 20-30 seconds under warm water to unmold, after which turn stick nicely to release.

Keto Cheese Pops – Low-Carb Popcorn

(Ready in about 8 mins :| Serving 1 | Difficulty: easy)

Per serving: kcal 88, Fat:7g, Net carbs:4g Protein:5g

Ingredients

- Hard cheese 100g

Instructions

1. Slice hard cheese into pieces first, and then into little squares.

2. Place it on a cookie sheet with a bakery release paper cover with the napkin.

3. Hold it on 48 hours in the kitchen.

4. Heat the oven until 200 c (392f)

5. Place the cheese inside the oven for three mins.

6. Enjoy your meal.

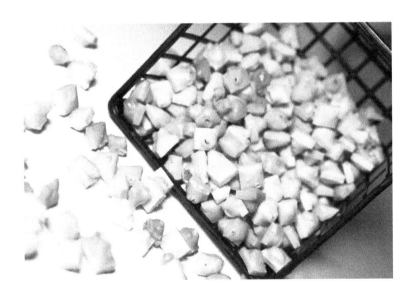

Dark Chocolate-Covered Walnuts

(Ready in about 30 mins| Serving 2 | Difficulty: easy)

Per serving kcal 160 Total Fat: 13g Net carbs:4.4g, Protein: 3g

Ingredients

- Shelled walnuts 2 cups
- Chocolate chopped unsweetened 4 oz
- Powdered Swerve sweetener ¼ cup
- Walnut oil 3 tbsp
- Vanilla extract ½ tsp
- Cocoa powder unsweetened 1 tbsp

Instructions

1. Line a cookie sheet with bakery release paper.

2. Combine the sugar, swerve powdered & almond oil/walnut Oil on low heat. Mix it until smooth & melted.

3. Whisk in the vanilla extract & Cocoa powder until smooth.

4. To thicken, let Cool for 5 mins.

5. Attach half of the walnuts & raise every walnut out from A fork, tap lightly on the surface to extract excessive coat.

6. Place every walnut mostly on the Ready cookie sheet. Repeat for Leftover walnuts.

7. Place the baking sheet 15-20 mins in the refrigerator.

8. If the coating begins thickening too much, gently Reheat to a little more liquid over low heat.

9. Work for a few walnuts at such a time, re-coating by falling again into the coating of chocolate and pulling out with a pick, pressing to extract any on foot.

10. Put on a cookie sheet, and chill Until solid in the fridge.

Mexican Hot Chocolate – Low-Carb and Gluten-Free

(Ready in about 10mins| Serving 20| Difficulty: very easy)

Per serving kcal 330, Total Fat: 31g Net carbs:3.8g, Protein: 7g

Ingredients

- Almond milk 1 ¼ cup
- Heavy cream ½ cup
- Cocoa powder gluten-free unsweetened 2 tbsp
- Swerve sweetener 1 tbsp
- Ground cinnamon ¼ tsp
- Chipotle powder 1/8-¼ tsp
- Whipped dollop cream & cinnamon sprinkle for garnish

Instructions

1. Mix almond milk, salt, chocolate powder, swerve, spice & chipotle powder into a med saucepan on normal heat.

2. Whisk together as good, after Which carries it to the simmer.

3. Remove it from fire, divide it B/w 2 mugs, & top it with cinnamon & chantilly cream.

4. Only apply a shot of good Coffee or espresso for an additional boost.

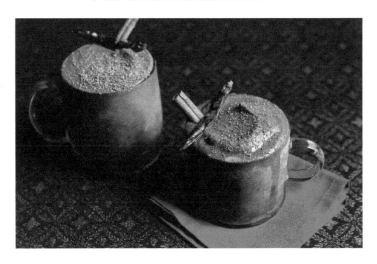

Homemade Thin Mints (Low-Carb and Gluten-Free)

(Ready in about 1hour| Serving 20 | Difficulty: easy)

Per serving: kcal 116, Fat: 10.4g, Net carbs:7g, Protein: 3g

Ingredients

Cookies:

- Almond Flour 1 3/4 cups
- Cocoa powder 1/3 cup
- Swerve sweetener 1/3 cup
- Baking powder 1 tsp
- Salt 1/4 tsp
- Slightly beaten large egg 1
- Butter melted 2 tbsp

- Vanilla extract 1/2 tsp

Coating:

- Coconut oil & butter1 tbsp
- Lily's dark chocolate 7 oz
- Peppermint extract 1 tsp

Instructions

Cookies:

1. Oven preheated to 300f, & Line 2 cookie sheets with bakery release paper
2. Combine the almond flour, cocoa sugar, sweetener, baking Soda/powder & salt in a big dish. Put the egg, butter as well as vanilla & stir it well until the dough fits in.
3. Roll out the dough b/w 2 pieces of bakery release Paper to optimal thickness but not more than one/four "wide. Take the parchment top Off and put aside.

4. Cut out dough circles using just a 2 inches diameter biscuit cutter and raise softly. Put biscuits on the ready cookie sheet. Pick up the dough and re-roll scraps till less can be left to roll out.

5. Bake cookies for 20-30 mins once it's strong to touch (this can differ based on how finely you roll the dough). Remove it and allow it to cool. They'll keep crisping up While they chill off.

Chocolate coating:

1. Put a bowl of metal over a pot of softly boiling water, stopping the bowl from entering the water. In a cup, melt the oil & chocolate, stirring until smooth. Mix in the peppermint Extract and clear from steam.

2. Dip the cookies into Cocoa, transform them over Using two forks and cover the cookie as a whole. Take the cookie out and tap the fork softly, mostly on the bowl's side, to remove the excess chocolate, after which put it on a waxed baking sheet with tape.

3. Refrigerate to Complete state.

Apple Cider Donut Bites

(Ready in about 30 mins| Serving 12 | Difficulty: easy)

Per serving: kcal 164, Fat: 13.7g, Net carbs:4.8g, Protein: 6.5g

Ingredients

Donut bites:

- Almond flour 2 cups
- Swerve sweetener 1/2 cup
- Whey protein powder unflavored 1/4 cup
- Baking powder 2 tsp
- Cinnamon 1/2 tsp
- Salt 1/2 tsp
- Large eggs 2
- Cup water 1/3

- Butter melted 1/4 cup
- Apple cider vinegar 1 1/2 tbsp
- Apple extract 1 1/2 tsp

Coating:

- Swerve sweetener 1/4 cup
- Cinnamon 1 to 2 tsp
- Butter melted 1/4 cup

Instructions

1. Oven Preheated to325f, then grease well a tiny muffin pan (use a standard muffin box with 24 cavities).
2. Mix all the almond meal, sweetener, protein powder, dried powder, spices & salt in the large bowl. Whisk until it's mixed in milk, sugar, butter, cider vinegar & apple extract.
3. Divide the mixture between the wells of the prepared tiny muffin pan. Bake for 15-20 mins, until the cupcakes are hard to touch. Remove &

allow it to cool for 10 mins, then Switch to the wire rack to completely cool.

4. Mix both sweetener & spices in a tiny bowl. Dip a full bite of donut in the softened butter, fully covering it. Then roll the combination into each donut snap.

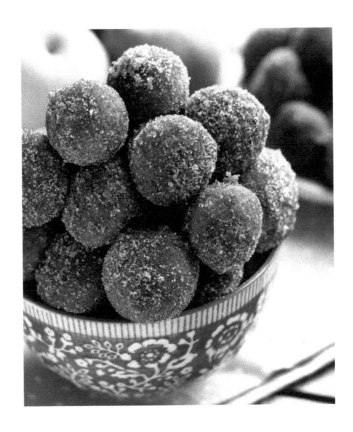

Low-Carb Almond Bark

(Ready in about 25 mins| Serving 20 | Difficulty: easy)

Per serving: kcal 144, Fat: 14g, Net carbs:5g, Protein: 3g

Ingredients

- Swerve sweetener 1/2 cup

- Water 2 tbsp

- Butter 1 tbsp

- Roasted almonds unsalted 1½ cups

- Sea salt ¼ tsp

- Cocoa butter 4 oz

- Chopped chocolate unsweetened 2.5 oz

- Powdered Swerve sweetener½ cup

- Cocoa powder ¾ cup

- Vanilla extract ½ tsp

- Additional Salt

Instructions

1. Line a big cookie sheet. Combine swerve & water in A med saucepan on med heat, stirring periodically. Put to a simmer, and steam for Around 7-9 mins before the mixture blacken. A combination is going to Smoke mildly, that's usual.

2. Remove the butter from the fire & whisk it. Attach the almonds & mix it to coat easily, then mix it in salt.

3. Place the almonds on the Cookie sheet set, splitting any clumps.

4. Melt the coconut butter & chocolate in A strong saucepan on med heat once smooth.

5. Add sifted erythritol powder, then Mix it in cocoa powder, until smooth.

6. Stir in the vanilla Extract and clear it from heat.

7. Reserve the almonds 1/4 Cup and set back. Stir in the Cocoa, the leftover almonds. Put over the same cookie sheet lined with parchment, Holding the nuts in such a single row.

8. Sprinkle with such an extra Estimated almond & sea salt.

9. Cool it.

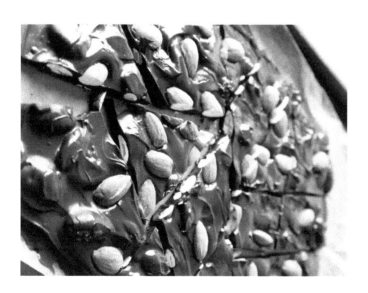

Keto Pistachio Truffles

(Ready in about 5 mins| Serving 1 | Difficulty: easy)

Per serving: kcal 121, Fat: 12g, Net carbs:0.5g, Protein: 1g

Ingredients

- Mascarpone cheese & softened 1 cup
- Pure vanilla extract 1/4 tsp
- Erythritol sweetener 3 tbsp
- Chopped pistachios 1/4 cup

Instructions

1. Mix the mascarpone, espresso, and sweetener into a tiny bowl.
2. Mix nicely with such a fork Either spatula, until fully mixed & smooth.
3. Place the pistacia vera on a small plate & roll the truffles onto them until they are coated fully.
4. Cool it for Thirty mins, then serve.
5. Place it in the freezer in an airtight jar for about 1 week.

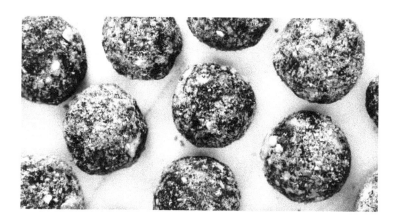

Keto Peanut Butter Cheesecake Bites

(Ready in about 30 mins| Serving 1 | Difficulty: easy)

Per serving: kcal 233, Fat: 22g, Net carbs:4g, Protein: 4g

Ingredients

- Cream cheese & softened 8 oz
- Powdered erythritol 1/4 cup
- Vanilla extract 1 tsp
- Heavy whipping cream 1/4 cup
- Peanut butter 1/4 cup
- Lily's sugar chocolate 3/4 cup
- Coconut oil 2 tsp

Instructions

1. Stir cream cheese, erythritol & Heavy cream until smooth.
2. Mix both peanut butter & vanilla Extract until completely blended, set aside.
3. Stir coconut Oil & melted chocolate.
4. Rub silicone cups with a mixture of chocolate & Put it in a refrigerator for five mins.
5. Repeat the last move & Freeze it for ten mins.
6. Put a few lbs of cheesecake fluff In a mug, then freeze it for fifteen mins.
7. Full cups of chocolate to fill soft cheesecake.
8. Put it in the fridge for about 1 hour.

Fat Bombs

(Ready in about 1hour 5mins| Serving 1 | Difficulty: easy)

Per serving: kcal 153, Fat: 16.6g, Net carbs:1.2g, Protein: 0.2g

Ingredients

- Coconut oil 1/2 cup
- Cacao butter 2 ounces
- Freeze-dried raspberries 1/2 cup
- Powdered erythritol sweetener 1/4 cup

Instructions

1. Top a twelve-cup muffin Tray with the liner material. Or use a muffin pan made of silicone.
2. In a medium saucepan, heat the coconut oil & cacao butter at low temperature until fully melted. Now Remove the heat from the pan.
3. In a mixing bowl, crush the freeze-dried strawberries.
4. Add sweetener &crushed berries to a saucepan. Mix until most of the sweetener dissolves.
5. Split the mixture into muffin cups. The strawberry powder falls to the floor — no problems. Only hold the mixture mixed as you push it into each mold, so there's some strawberry powder on top.
6. Refrigerate for one hr Until it's strong. They can keep over Several weeks in the fridge.

Cheesy Pottery Zucchini (Vegetarian Café)

(Ready in about 50 minutes | Difficulty: easy |Servings 4)

Per serving; kcal 155, 12.9 g Fat; 3.5 g Carbs; 0.8 g fibre; 7.6 g Protein; 0.2 g

Ingredients:

- Non-stick cooking spray
- 2 cups of zucchini,
- 2 tablespoons leeks thinly diced,
- 1/2 teaspoon salt
- Freshly ground black pepper,
- 1/2 teaspoon dried basil to taste
- 1/2 tablespoon of dried oregano
- 1/2 cup Cheddar cheese grated,

- 1/4 cup of heavy cream

- 4 Tablespoons Parmesan cheese,

- 1 tablespoon butter freshly grated,

Instructions:

1. Preheat the oven to 370 degrees F. Grease a saucepan gently. Use a non-stick mist for cooking. Add 1 tablespoon of new Garlic, hazelnuts. Place 1 cup of the slices of zucchini in the dish; add 1 spoonful of leeks; sprinkle Season with oil, basil, pepper, and oregano. Finish Cheddar cheese with 1/4 cup. Echo the layers once again. Whisk the heavy cream in a mixing dish with Parmesan, butter, and Garlic. Break this combination over the layer of zucchini and the layers of Cheese.

2. Position in the preheated furnace and cook to the outside for around 40 to 45 minutes until the edges are beautifully browned. Spray with chopped chives, if required.

Chocolate Chip Cookie Dough Bites

(Ready in about 25 minutes | Serving 24 | Difficulty: easy)

Per serving: kcal 110, Fat: 10g, Net carbs:2g, Protein:2g

Ingredients

Cookie dough bites

- Almond flour 2 cups
- Confectioner's swerve sweetener 1/2 cup
- Salt 1/4 tsp
- Melted butter 6 tbsp
- Vanilla extract 1 tsp
- Chocolate chips sugar-free 1/3 cup

Instructions

1. Oven preheated to 300f & line a 9 X 9 inches pan with bakery release paper.
2. Mix the coconut, peanuts, pecan, & Seeds of sunflowers in the food processor. Heat on high until the combination resembles finely textured crumbs.
3. Shift it to a bowl & Mix in the chocolate morsels, cranberries & salt.
4. Melt butter with yacon or even the Fiber syrup in a med saucepan on low heat. When molten, stir until Smooth in powdered sweetener. Place the Vanilla extract in.
5. In the nut/coconut mixture, Whisk your butter mixture until completely mixed. Push uniformly into the ready Baking pan at the rim. To further press it down & compress it as far as possible, have used the flat-bottomed bottle or measurement cup.
6. Bake for twenty-five min, or until the sides become golden brown. Let it cool down entirely within the pan, after which take them out through parchment. Use a fine knife to Cut these into bars.

Cookie Teapots

1. Mix all the almond meal, the Swerve confectioners, and salt in a big bowl. Mix Softened butter & vanilla extract as well as mix in chocolate morsels.
2. Scoop the dough out through curved tbsp & press a couple of times into your palm to help keep it together, then shape it into a ball. Put on a baking sheet lined with Waxed paper & repeat it with leftover dough.
3. If you want, you should stop here Because these are fine as they are. But placing the baking sheet in the refrigerator for one hour.

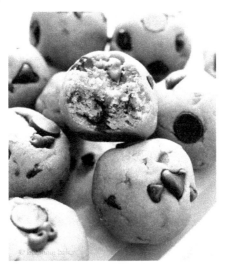

Keto Cinnamon Butter Cookies Recipe

(Ready in about 30mins| Serving 1 | Difficulty: easy)

Per serving: kcal 146, Fat: 14g, Net carbs:1g, Protein:4g

Ingredients

- Almond meal 2 cups

- Salted butter 1/2 cup

- Egg 1

- Vanilla extract 1 tsp

- Ground cinnamon 1 tsp

- Liquid stevia 1 tsp

Instructions

1. The oven preheated about 300F.

2. In the mixing bowl, stir all the components, and blend until just mixed.

3. Roll in fifteen balls & put on a tray of a greased baking sheet.

4. Put in the microwave, bake it for five mins.

5. Cut the
   dough with such a fork and push it hard.

6. Move to oven & cook for 18-20 mins.

7. Let cool it for five mins.

Dark Chocolate Fudgsicles

(Ready in about 8hours 25 mins| Serving 6 | Difficulty: medium)

Per serving: kcal 133, Fat: 14g, Net carbs:3g, Protein:1g

Ingredients

- Coconut milk 13.5 oz

- Cocoa powder 1/4 cup

- Erythritol 1/4 cup

- Stevia glycerite 6 drops

- Xanthan gum rounded 1/8 tsp

Instructions

1. Put everything in a saucepan except stevia & xanthan gum, then brings to a boil. Put Down warmth to maintain it. Make sure that erythritol dissolves & boil to bloom that cocoa powder for fifteen mins.
2. To adjust the flavor of your preference, Apply two drops of stevia glycerite at a time.
3. Put the xanthan gum in your blender & Gently distribute it all over the heated fudgsicle mixture. Stir strongly until It significantly gets thicker. That must be consistent with Chocolate pudding. This is the move stopping a fudgsicles from becoming rock hard in the refrigerator.
4. Cool the blend & Split it into the popsicle mold. Freeze for 8 hrs or longer, and ideally overnight.

Keto Cheese Straws

(Ready in about 50 mins| Serving 48 | Difficulty: easy)

Per serving: kcal 209, Fat: 18.6g, Net carbs:4.5g, Protein:6.3g

Ingredients

- Almond flour 1 ¾ cup

- Coconut flour 2 tbsp

- Salt ¾ tsp

- Xanthan gum ½ tsp

- Garlic powder ½ tsp

- Cayenne optional ¼-½ tsp

- Chopped butter ½ cup

- Sharp cheddar grated 4 ounces

- Egg yolk 1

Instructions

1. Oven preheated to 300f, & line 2 cookie sheet with bake ry release paper.

2. In a food processor, place the almond meal, Coconut fl our, salt, xanthan gum, garlic powder & cayenne. Pulse a couple of times to mix.

3. Sprinkle the butter bits and the grated cheese over. The dry products, then apply the yolk of the egg. Pulse until the dough is fully mixed, then collect it into a ball.

4. Move the dough to an open star tip-fitted Piping bag & pipe your dough into three inches rows. They could be quite tight Together because they're not expanding. (then you can bring your dough to the cookie press & make enjoyable shapes).

5. Bake for 20-25 minutes until golden brown, then stop your oven & let the straws stay inside for another five mins. Keep a keen watch on them, so that they wouldn't get too much brown.

6. Remove from the pan & let it cool fully.

Everything Bagel Cucumber Bites

(Ready in about 25 mins| Serving 8 | Difficulty: medium)

Per serving: kcal 93, Fat: 7.9g, Net carbs: 2.7g, Protein: 1.5g

Ingredients

Everything bagel seasoning:

- Poppy seeds 1 tsp

- Sesame seeds 1 tsp

- Dried minced garlic 1/2 tsp

- Dried minced onion 1/2 tsp

- Crushed caraway seeds 1/4 tsp

- Coarse salt 1/4 tsp

Cucumber bites:

- Medium cucumber 1

- Cream cheese 4 ounces

- Butter softened 2 tbsp

- Greek yogurt 2 tbsp

- Garlic powder 1/2 tsp

- Salt 1/4 tsp

Instructions

Everything bagel seasoning:

1. Whisk all of the
   ingredients with Each other in a bowl. Place On asi
   de.

Cucumber Snacks:

1. Use a fine knife to Cut off the cucumber. Cross-slice
   that cucumber into 1/4 "thick Pieces & placed on
   the platter.

2. Hit the cream cheese, butter, milk, garlic powder & salt in a med bowl until they are well mixed and smooth.
3. Attach a star-shaped tip to the piping bag & Fill the bag with a combination of cream cheese. Decoratively pouring the Cucumber slices on top.
4. Sprinkle with all bagel seasoning on every slice and serve

Homemade Chicharrones

(Ready in about 3hours 50 mins:| Serving 1 | Difficulty: easy)

Per serving: kcal 152, Fat: 9g, Protein:17g

Ingredients

- Pork back fat & skin 3-5 lbs.

- Extra cooking oil

- Sea salt-taste

- Pepper-taste

Instructions

1. Oven preheated to 250f & set A rack of wire over a cookie sheet.

2. Cut pork skin & fat into long strips, around 2 inches wide, using a keen knife. Score the fat every 2 Inches on every stripe. Insert the knife carefully on 1 end of the strip between the skin & fat, then removes a portion of fat.

3. Once that first part of fat has been erased, it can hold the skin in 1 Hand while sliding a knife down the strip to remove most of the fat. Once more, a little bit of fat that still clings to the skin is fine.

4. Cut each stripe into two-inch squares & put, fat-side down, on wire rack whenever the fat has been removed.

5. In the meantime, if you want to cook the chicharrones with the pork fat, place them in the large saucepan on med heat. Cook gently, about 2 hrs, until most of the fat has liquified. This is also the way you could even render lard besides future use in cooking. To remove the remaining Solids, choose a slotted spoon.

6. When the baking time is up, heat oil/lard into the pan to a depth of 1/3. Or you can have just a few other inches of oil & cook the pork rinds in lots. Oil must be hot, but it should not bubble.

7. Add pork rinds & cook it for about 3-5 Mins, until they bubble & puff up. Erase & sink onto a towel-lined sheet of paper. Instantly sprinkle with salt & pepper.

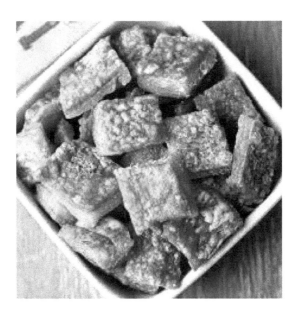

Keto Cheddar Jalapeno Meatballs

(Ready in about 45 mins:| Serving 8 | Difficulty: easy)

Per serving: kcal 368, Fat: 24g, Net carbs:1.1g Protein:33.4g

Ingredients

- Ground beef 1 ½ lbs.

- Sharp cheddar grated 6 ounces

- Pork rind crumbs ½ cup

- Large egg 1

- Large jalapeno diced

- Chopped cilantro 2 tbsp

- Chili powder 1 tsp

- Garlic powder 1 tsp

- Salt 1 tsp

- Cumin ½ tsp

- Pepper ½ tsp

Instructions

1. Oven preheated to 375 & line the Bakery release paper with a big rimmed cookie sheet.
2. Mix all the ingredients into the A bowl of a big food processor. A process on high until excellently combined, scraping Away from the processor's sides as needed.
3. Alternatively, you can mix everything by hand in a bowl. To form a cohesive mixture, genuinely working the ingredients together.
4. Roll into 1½-inch balls and place on the ready cookie sheet about 1 inch apart. Bake for twenty mins, Till cooked & browned.
5. Serve warm.

Taco Bites (Mini)

(Ready in about 35 mins:| Serving 32 | Difficulty: easy)

Per serving: kcal 329, Fat: 22.15g, Net carbs:3.1g Protein:25.2g

Ingredients

- Ground beef grass-fed O organics 1 lb.

- O organics melted salted butter 2 tbsp.

- Taco seasoning 3 tbsp

- Large egg 1

- O organics shredded cheese Mexican blend 6 ounces

- Salsa O organics 1 cup

- Other garnish

Instructions

1. In a wide skillet on med heat, the meat is sauteed, separating the Clumps by using the

wooden spoon, until nearly cooked through. Add seasoning to the taco & Proceed to sauté until thoroughly cooked. Take off heat & allow it to cool.

2. To 350F, preheat the oven and spray the butter (melted) with a decent nonstick tiny muffin cup. This recipe produces about thirty-two tiny muffins, so if more than 1 mini muffin tray you don't have, you can need to operate in batches.

3. Beat the eggs into a big bowl. Add taco meat & the Grilled cheese on 4 ounces. Mix it completely.

4. Sprinkle with the leftover melted cheese & muffin cups are filled to around 3⁄4 complete. Bake for 15-20 mins, until puffed to touch & strong. Remove, and allow to cool for ten mins. Using a small, lightweight spatula to Pass along the side to release muffins.

5. Serve taco toppings include sauce, sour cream & guacamole for your pick.

Stuffed Baby Peppers

(Ready in about 10 mins | Serving 4-6 | Difficulty: easy)

Per serving 28kcal, fat: 2g, protein: 1g

Ingredients

- Baby peppers

- Cream cheese

Instructions

1. Clean every baby pepper and cut the top off, scooping out any little seeds that might exist.

2. Slowly stuff every pepper with cream cheese with a fine knife before they are finished.

3. Place in the refrigerator for up to three days.

Spanakopita Hand Pies

(Ready in about 40 mins:| Serving 16 | Difficulty: easy)

Per serving: kcal 123, Fat: 9.5g, Net carbs:3.4g
Protein:5.6g

Ingredients

- Spinach thawed frozen 6 ounces

- Crumbled feta cheese 1 cup

- Large egg 1

- Chopped onion 1/4 cup

- Garlic minced 1 clove

- Salt 3/4 tsp

- Pepper 1/2 tsp

- Mozzarella dough 1

- Extra almond flour to roll out.

Instructions

1. Oven Preheated to 350F.

2. Put the spinach in a dish towel & force the extra moisture out. Shift to Wide bowl. Add the feta, potato, cabbage, garlic, salt, & pepper, then mix until good.

3. Sprinkle any 2 to 3 tsp of almond flour on a work surface. Roll the dough out to around sixteen inches by sixteen inches in a wide rectangle. Cut it into sixteen equal squares using such a sharp knife or a pizza cutter.

4. Place around one spinach combination tbsp into the middle of each rectangle. Roll the dough square diagonally over to create a pastry formed like a triangle. When the dough splits or

falls as it bends, easily pinch back & shape across the filling.

5. Put the triangles on a prepared cookie sheet & create a small slit only at the top of each to make the steam to exit. Bake until golden brown, For 20 mins. Remove from the skillet & let it cool.

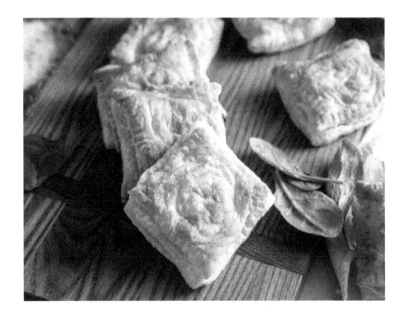

Keto Buffalo Chicken Sausage Balls

(Ready in about 40 mins:| Serving 12 | Difficulty: easy)

Per serving: kcal 255, fat: 14.02g, Net carbs: 3.90g Protein:14.5g

Sausage balls Ingredients

- Chicken sausage 24 ounces

- Cheddar cheese 1 cup shredded

- Almond flour 1 cup

- Coconut flour 3 tbsp

- Sauce buffalo wing 1/2 cup

- Salt 1 tsp

- Pepper ½ tsp

- Cayenne 1/2 tsp

Dipping sauce bleu cheese ranch:

- Mayonnaise cup 1/3

- Almond milk unsweetened 1/3 cup

- Garlic minced 2 cloves

- Dried parsley ½ tsp

- Dried dill 1 tsp

- Pepper ½ tsp

- Salt ½ tsp

- Cheese crumbled bleu ¼ cup

Instructions

Balls Sausage:

1. To 350F, preheat the oven and line 2 wide cookie sheets with bakery release paper.

2. Combine the bacon, cheddar cheese, buffalo sauce, coconut flour, almond flour, cayenne salt, and pepper in a wide dish. Combine completely.

3. Roll into balls, one inch & put on prepared sheet for baking around an inch apart. Bake for 25 mins until it becomes golden brown.

Dipping sauce:

1. In a medium dish, add mayonnaise, garlic, dill, almond milk, parsley, pepper, and salt. Then stir and blend with cheese crumbled bleu.

Keto Rosemary Parmesan Crackers

(Ready in about 1hour 10 mins:| Serving 10 | Difficulty: easy)

Per serving: kcal 179, Fat: 15.1g, Net carbs:5.6g, Protein:8.5g

Ingredients

- Sunflower seed flour 2 cups

- Finely grated parmesan 3/4 cup

- Fresh rosemary chopped 2 tbsp

- Garlic powder 1/2 tsp

- Baking powder 1/2 tsp

- Salt 1/2 tsp

- Large egg 1

- Melted butter 2 tbsp

- Coarse salt for sprinkling

Instructions

1. Oven Preheated to 300F.

2. Combine the seed flour of sunflower, parmesan, rosemary, ginger, baking powder/soda & salt in a large dish.

3. Mix within butter & egg before the dough falls around.

4. Turn the dough out & pat it into the harsh rectangle onto a broad silicone cookie sheet. Using a large sheet of Bakery release paper on the cover. Stretch out to a thickness of around 1/4-1/8 inches. Put the Parchment aside.

5. To grade into 2-inch pieces, use a fine knife or pizza wheel. Sprinkle the Sea salt. Move to a broadsheet of a cookie sheet.

6. Bake 40-45 mins, or until the sides are golden brown & the crackers are solid if touch. Remove

and let it cool down before breaking up entirely. They'll keep crisping Up while they cool.

7. The
recipe generates around 40 crackers, based on how finely the dough is rolled.

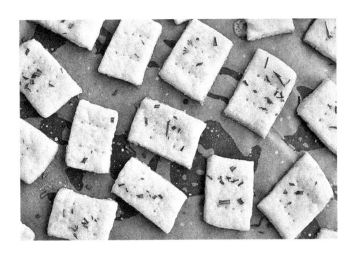

Low-Carb Pepperoni Pizza Bites

(Ready in about 18 mins:| Serving 24 | Difficulty: easy)

Per serving: kcal 81, Fat: 6g, Net carbs: 1g Protein: 5g

Ingredients

- Pepperoni 24 slices

- Small basil leaves 24

- Pizza sauce small 1 jar

- Mozzarella balls 24 mini

Instructions

1. Oven preheated to 400F. Snip four 1/2-inch cut-outs along the sides of Each pepperoni slice using kitchen shears,

leaving the middle uncut. Per pepperoni will appear Like a circular arrow.

2. Push down every pepperoni into a tiny muffin tin. Bake until the sides are crispy for 5-6 Mins; however, the pepperoni is always hot. Let allow the pepperoni chill within pans to crisp for 5 mins, so they retain their form. Then transfer the cups onto a lined sheet of paper towel to extract excess liquid.

3. Wipe the oil with a towel out of the muffin Tray, after which return the cups to the tray. In the bottom of each cup, put a tiny basil leaf, accompanied by 1 Tsp of pizza sauce, a small mozzarella nut, as well as an olive slice.

4. Return to the oven for two-three mins Before the cheese begins to melt. Allow the cups for 3- 5 mins to chill more before serving.

Pickle Rollups

(Ready in about 12 mins:| Serving 4 | Difficulty: easy)

Per serving: kcal 286, Fat: 26g, Net carbs:4g Protein:10g

Ingredients

- Corned beef lunch meat 8 slices

- Softened cream cheese 4 oz

- Dill pickles 4 med

Instructions

1. Place corned beef on a rough surface in the stacks of 2.

2. Place one ounce of cream Cheese over each stack. Put a pickle Right in each middle. Roll the corned beef across the pickles, then split into 4 equal pieces per slice.

Two Ingredient Cheese Crisps

(Ready in about 22 mins:| Serving 1 | Difficulty: easy)

Per serving: kcal 82, Fat: 6g, Net carbs:1g Protein:6g

Ingredients

- Shredded cheese 1 cup

- Egg whites only 2

Instructions

1. Oven Preheated to 400.

2. Mix the white egg, cheddar, & any Herbs/spice s into a tiny bowl.

3. Grease a twenty-four slot mini muffin tray into muffin tins & drop very tiny parts of the cheese mixture.

4. Spread it out,
   making it as thin to keep it crispy.

5. Bake it for 10-20 mins.

6. Let It cool before eating.

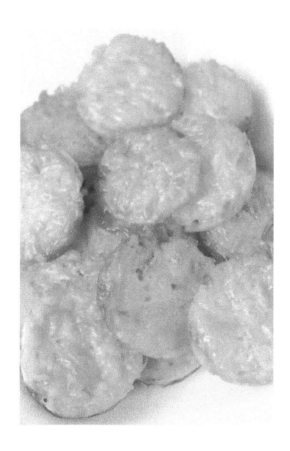

Low-Carb Pinwheels with Bacon and Cream Cheese

(Ready in about 15 mins:| Serving 10 | Difficulty: easy)

Per serving: kcal 143, Fat: 12g, Net carbs:2g Protein:6g

Ingredients

- Ham 18 slices

- Bacon cooked 5 to 8 slices

- Cream cheese 4 oz

- Ranch seasoning 1-1/2

- Chopped black olives ¼ cup

Instruction

1. Put the salami/ham down into 4x2 Alternating rows on a cutting board.

2. Spread the salami over the cream cheese. If the cream cheese becomes too hard to apply with a knife, you may attempt to arrange It b/w 2 wax paper sheets & roll it out with a rolling pin, then bring it on the salami or ham.

3. Sprinkle the cream cheese on the Ranch seaso ning, then apply the black olives.

4. Shortly place your slices of bacon over the cream cheese.

5. Turn the pinwheels slowly long side- long side, spinning as stiffly as possible.

6. Securely keep the roll, then break it into 1- 2 "parts.

7. Use as an appetizer, or individually package each portion with a greaseproof paper for single servings.

Keto Soft Pretzel

(Ready in about 29 mins:| Serving 6 | Difficulty: easy)

Per serving: kcal 449, Fat: 35.5g, Net carbs: 10g, Protein:27.8g

Ingredients

- Baking powder 1tbsp

- Garlic powder 1tbsp

- Onion powder 1 tbsp

- Large egg 3

- Shredded mozzarella cheese 3 cups

- Cream cheese 5 tbsp

- Salt for topping

Instructions

1. Oven preheated to 425 °. Line a rimmed cookie sheet with bakery release paper.

2. Add the almond flour/meal, baking powder/soda, garlic powder & onion powder in a med bowl. Blend until it's combined.

3. Smash 1 of the eggs in a tiny bowl & fork whisk. It would be the wash of the egg for the top of the pretzels as well as the other 2 eggs for the dough.

4. Add mozzarella cheese & cream cheese in a big microwave safe blending bowl. Microwave it for One min and 30 sec. Now remove it from the microwave & blend to mix.

5. Apply the remaining two eggs & the mixture of almond flour to the mixing bowl. Combine until all ingredients are fully mixed. If The dough becomes too

stringy and impracticable, just place it back in the oven for 30 seconds to loosen & continue to blend.

6. Split the dough into six equal parts. Roll each piece into a large, thin piece that resembles a breadstick. Fold each piece into the form of a pretzel.

7. Rub the egg wash Over the top within each pretzel.

8. Brush over the surface with coarse sea salt.

9. Bake 12 to 14 Mins on a center rack.

Fathead Sausage Rolls

(Ready in about 45 mins:| Serving 6 | Difficulty: easy)

Per serving: kcal 470, Fat: 39.1g, Net carbs:3.6g
Protein:26g

Ingredients

- Sausages 500 g

- Onion flakes to garnish

Fathead pastry

- Grated mozzarella 170 g

- 85 g almond meal/flour

- Cream cheese 2 tbsp

- Egg 1

- Pinch salt

- Onion flakes 1 tsp

Instructions

Pre-cook the sausages

1. Using
   a fine knife, cut your sausage casing down the
   middle. Peel the wrapping back.

2. Put every sausage on even A lined oven tray
   & cook for ten mins at 180c/350f.

Fat Pastry head

1. Bake the fat head Pastry while frying the
   sausages.

2. In a microwave cup, put together the
   shredded/grated cheese and the almond
   flour/meal. Add your cream cheese. Now
   microwave it for one minute.

3. Then pulse over high for a thirty sec. Detach
   and mix Again. Add the flakes of onion, salt &
   egg.

4. Put your fat head pastry b/w two pieces of Bakery release paper & roll into a small, rectangular bowl.

5. Cut your fat head pastry on one side & put the Sausages around the edge. Start rolling it, then cut off the excessive pastry.

6. Slice Into sausage rolls & drizzle/spray the oil over the end. Sprinkle with flakes of onion to garnish.

7. Bake for 12 to 15 minutes at 220c/425f, until it's crispy all over.

Salt and Vinegar Zucchini Chips

(Ready in about 12hours 15 mins:| Serving 8 | Difficulty: easy)

Per serving: kcal 40, Fat: 3.6g, Net carbs: 2.9g Protein: 0.7g

Ingredients

- Thinly sliced zucchini 4 cups

- Additional virgin olive oil 2 tbsp

- White balsamic vinegar 2 tbsp

- Sea salt 2 tsp

Instructions

1. Using an as small as Possible mandolin or a slice of zucchini.

2. Mix the olive oil & Vinegar in a tiny bowl together.

3. In a wide bowl, put the zucchini, and mix it with oil & vinegar.

4. Add the zucchini to the dehydrating In even layers & sprinkle it with the coarse salt.

5. The drying period would differ based on how thin you cut the zucchini and the dehydrator, anywhere from 8 to 14 hrs. I set the temperature of 135F.

6. Line the baking sheet with bakery release paper in the oven. Spread the zucchini uniformly. Bake around 200 degrees f for 2 to 3 hrs.

7. The chips are placed inside an airtight jar.

Cheesy Bacon Zucchini Skins

(Ready in about 20 mins:| Serving 12 | Difficulty: easy)

Per serving: kcal 127, Fat: 11g, Net carbs:2g Protein:4g

Ingredients

- Bacon 6 slices

- Zucchini 3 medium

- Monterey jack cheese chopped 1 cup

- Green onions sliced 3

- Sour cream 1 cup

Instruction

1. Chop the bacon & sauté over med heat in a frying pan until crispy, drain it on towels.

84

2. Break the zucchini lengthwise in two. Split in half and slice off each zucchini's ends, making four skins, comprising twelve skins.

3. Using a wide spoon, scoop tightly out the white portion of the zucchini leaving around 1/4 "within the skins. Remove the interior of the zucchini and put the skins cut side up on a large baking sheet.

4. Scatter with cheese & crumbled bacon uniformly. Bake for 5 to 10 mins at 400 degrees or until the cheese is finished and the zucchini is somewhat soft (they can always have a little crunch).

5. Before topping with green onion, let it chill for 5 mins and serve it with sour cream/ranch dressing to dip.

Bacon Jalapeño Cheese Ball

(Ready in about 2hour 10 mins:| Serving 1 | difficulty: easy)

Per serving: kcal 110, Fat: 9g, Net carbs:2g Protein:4g

Ingredients

- Softened cream cheese 1 8 ounce

- Jalapeño diced chopped 5 tbsp

- Cooked bacon divided ☐ cup

- Garlic salt ¾ tsp

- Liquid smoke ¼ tsp

Instructions

1. Combine milk softened cheese with 3 tsp jalapeno, one/three cup bacon, garlic salt & liquid smoke in a med bowl.

2. Shape into a ball, cover in plastic wrap, and cool down for 2 hours.

3. Now remove the cheese ball from plastic wrap & roll onto the leftover jalapenos & crumbled bacon to cover.

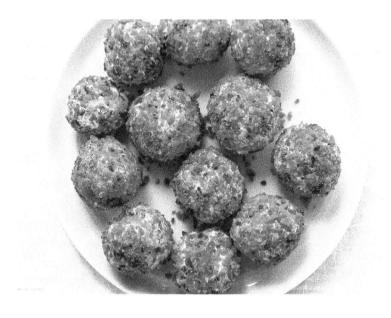

Low-Carb Everything Crackers

(Ready in about 50 mins:| Serving 36 | Difficulty: easy)

Per serving: kcal 212, fat: 17.1, Net carbs:5.8g Protein:8.1g

Ingredients

- Large egg

- Garlic powder 1/2 ts

- Onion Powder 1/2 tsp

- Kosher Salt 1/4 tsp

- Bagel seasoning 2 tbsp

- Fine almond flour 1&3/4 cups

Instructions

1. Oven preheated to 350f. Mix the seasoning bagel's 1 tbsp, egg, garlic powder, onion powder & salt.

2. Add the almond flour and blend until it forms a pastry. Flatten among 2 sheets of bakery release paper or even on a waxed paper and a Silpat. Spread out to a thickness of 1/8.

3. Sprinkle with the waxed paper on the remaining spoonful of bagel seasoning and press into bread.

4. Use a knife or pizza cutter to cut into squares.

5. Directly transfer parchment or Silpat to the baking sheet.

6. Cook 10 minutes. Test to see if brown is cooked in golden color. If not, so put another 2 minutes.

Peanut Butter Granola

(Ready in about 40 mins | serving 12 | Difficulty: easy)

Per serving: kcal 338, fat: 30.08g, net carbs: 9.74g, Protein: 9.36g

Ingredients

- Almonds 1 1/2 cups

- Pecans 1 1/2 cups

- Almond flour or shredded coconut 1 cup

- Sunflower seeds 1/4 cup

- Swerve sweetener 1/3 cup

- Collagen protein powder or vanilla whey protein powder 1/3 cup

- Peanut butter 1/3 cup

- Butter 1/4 cup

- Water 1/4 cup

Instructions

1. Oven preheated to 300f & line a large baking paper with a covered baking tray.
2. In the mixing bowl, process the almonds and pecans with larger pieces until they resemble-fine scraps. Mix in chopped nuts, sweetener, sunflower seeds & vanilla whey protein and transfer it to the large bowl.
3. Evaporate peanut butter & butter together in a non - stick frying pan.
4. Place melted peanut butter over a mixture of nut and mix excellently, tossing lightly.
5. Mix the mixture. Combination clumps around each other.
6. Spread the mixture evenly over the ready baking sheet & bake for 30 mins, mixing through halfway. Remove, and allow it to cool.

Keto Salted Caramel Hot Chocolate

(Ready in about 6 mins | serving 1 | difficulty: easy)

Per serving: kcal 210, Fat: 16g, net carbs: 4.5g, Protein: 14.4g

Ingredients

- Hemp milk or unsweetened almond 1/2 cup

- Heavy whipping cream 2 tablespoon

- Cocoa powder 1 tbsp

- Salted caramel collagen 1-2 tbsp

- Liquid or powdered sweetener

- (optional) whipped cream lightly sweetened

- (optional) caramel sauce sugar-free

Instructions

1. In a small saucepan over medium heat, combine the almond or hemp milk and the heavy cream. Bring it to a simmer.

2. Add the cocoa powder and collagen to a blender. Pour in the hot milk and blend until frothy. Taste and adjust for sweetness.

3. Top with lightly sweetened whipped cream and some homemade caramel sauce to take it over the top

Keto Brownie Bark

(Ready in about 45 mins | serving 12 | Difficulty: medium)

Per serving: kcal 98, Fat: 8.3g, net carbs: 4.3g, Protein: 2.4g

Ingredients

- Almond flour 1/2 cup
- Baking powder 1/2 tsp
- Salt 1/4 tsp
- Egg whites 2 large
- Swerve sweetener granular 1/2 cup
- Cocoa powder 3 tbsp
- Instant coffee (optional) 1 tsp
- Butter melted 1/4 cup
- Heavy whipping cream 1 tbsp
- Vanilla 1/2 tsp
- Chocolate chips sugar-free 1/3 cups

Instructions

1. Oven preheated to 325f, and line a baking sheet with bakery release paper. Greaseproof paper to the bakery release paper.

2. Stir together all the baking powder, almond powder as well as salt in the small bowl.

3. Beat a white egg in the large mixing bowl until they're frothy. Beat until smooth in cocoa powder, sweetener & instant coffee, after which beat in softened butter, vanilla & cream. Beat in a mixture of almond meal until it's combined.

4. Spread batter over nonstick baking paper in a 12 by 8-inch rectangle. Stir the chocolate morsels.

5. Bake and set for 18 mins, until puffed. Now remove it from the oven and turn off the Oven and allow to cool for 15 mins.

6. To cut it into 2inch squares, use a filet knife or pizza cutter but don't separate. Return it to a hot oven for 8-10 mins to gently crisp up.

7. Remove, allow it cool down & then split it into squares.

Homemade Nutella Sugar-Free

(Ready in about 20 mins | serving 6 | Difficulty: easy)

Per serving: kcal 158, fat: 18.23g, net carbs: 4.74g, Protein: 3.33g

Ingredients

- Hazelnuts toasted & husked 3/4 cup

- Melted coconut oil or avocado oil 2-3 tbsp

- Cocoa powder 2 tbsp

- Powdered Swerve sweetener 2 tbsp

- Vanilla extract 1/2 tsp

- Pinch salt

Instructions

1. Crush hazelnuts in a mixing bowl or a full power blender until deftly ground & start clumping together.

2. Add two spoonfuls of oil & continue to whip until the nuts become smooth in the butter. Add rest of the ingredients, then mix until well mashed. If the combination is quite thick, then add an extra table cubic oil.

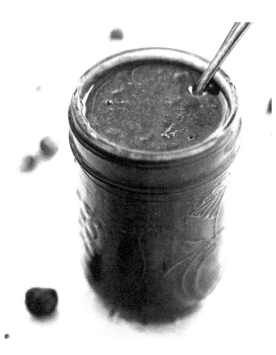

Snickerdoodle Truffles

(Ready in about 20 mins | serving 12 | Difficulty: easy)

Per serving: kcal 150, Fat: 14g, net carbs: 13g, Protein: 3g

Ingredients

- Almond flour 2 cups

- Swerve, confectioners 1/2 cup

- Tartar cream 1 tsp

- Ground cinnamon 1 tsp

- Salt 1/4 tsp

- Butter melted 6 tbsp

- Vanilla extract 1 tsp

Instructions

Truffles

1. Mix almond powder, swerve, tartar cream, cinnamon & salt in the large bowl. Incorporate softened butter & vanilla extract until the dough gets together. If dough becomes too crumbly to scrape together, add a spoonful of water & stir it.

2. Scoop out dough through the circular tablespoon and press just a few times in your palm to help hold it together. After this, shape it into a ball. Put on a baking tray lined with paraffin paper & repeat it with existing dough.

Low-Carb & Gluten-Free Coconut Chocolate Chip Cookies

(ready in about 30 mins | serving 20 cookies | Difficulty: easy)

Per serving: kcal 238, fat: 21.59g, net carbs: 8.18g, Protein: 4.39g

Ingredients

- Almond Flour 1 1/4 cups

- Unsweetened coconut finely shredded 3/4 cups

- Baking powder 1 tsp

- Salt 1/2 tsp

- Butter softened 1/2 cup

- Swerve sweetener 1/2 cup

- Yacon syrup 2 tsp

- Vanilla extract 1/2 tsp

- Large egg 1

- Chocolate chips sugar-free 1/3 cup

Instructions

1. Oven preheated to 325f, & line the large parchment or polyurethane liner cooking sheet.
2. Whisk the almond powder, cocoa powder, baking soda as well as salt with each other in a mixing bowl.
3. Softened butter with the molasses & erythritol in the large bowl. In vanilla & egg beat until just combined. Hit through flour mixture until it's mixed with dough. Mix in free of sugar chocolate morsels or hand - made chocolate-free chips
4. Shape the dough into the 1/2inch pieces and put it on a cookie sheet 2-inch apart, push every ball to 2 1/2inch thick with the heel of one's hand.
5. Bake twelve to fifteen mins, until just brown & hardly firm to touch.
6. Remove it from the oven and allow the pan to cool.

Peanut Butter & Jam Cups

(Ready in about 15 mins | serving 12 |Difficulty: easy)

Per serving: kcal 223, Fat: 14g, net carbs:4.5g, Protein:3.9g

Ingredients

- Raspberries ¾ c up
- Water 1/4 cup
- Powdered Swerve sweetener 6-8 tbsp
- Grass-fed gelatin 1 tsp
- Creamy peanut butter 3/4 cup
- Coconut oil 3/4 cup

Instructions

1. Use twelve polysiloxanes to line the baking tray.
2. Merge the raspberries & water in the medium saucepan over med heat. Bring it to boil & turn down the heat & simmer for five min. Mash a spoon on lingonberry.

3. Stir the powder form sweetener in 2 -4 mix in grass-fed gelatine & allow the peanut-butter combination to cool when it is being prepared.
4. Blend peanut oil & copra oil in a mixing bowl. Cook 30-60 second on high, until melted. Whisk powder form sweetener in 2–4 tbsp.
5. Divide half of its peanut oil mixture into the twelve cups and set about 15 minutes in the refrigerator to get firm. Split the raspberry mixture into cups & top it with the remaining butter peanut mixture.
6. Cool until it becomes firm

Classic Blueberry Scones

(Ready in about 40 mins | serving 12 | Difficulty: easy)

Per serving: kcal 153, Fat: 12.5g, net carbs:7.21g, Protein:5.55g

Ingredients

- Almond flour 2 cups
- Swerve sweetener 1/3 cup
- Coconut flour 1/4 cup
- Baking powder 1 tbsp
- Salt 1/4 tsp
- Large eggs 2
- Whipping cream 1/4 cup
- Vanilla extract 1/2 tsp
- Fresh blueberries 3/4 cup

Instructions

1. To 325F, preheat the oven and line with parchment a big baking sheet or silicone lining

2. Whisk the sweetener, almond flour, baking powder, coconut flour, and salt together in a big pot.

3. Add the eggs, mixing the cream and the vanilla, then blend until the dough starts to fit. Attach the blueberries, then function through the dough carefully.

4. Assemble the dough and transfer to the baking dish. Pat into a 10 x 8-inch rectangle.

5. Using a big, sharp knife to cut in 6 squares. Then diagonally split one of those squares into 2 triangles. Pick the scones softly and scatter them across the oven.

6. Bake for 20-25 mins, until brown (golden) and firm it should be. Remove and allow to cool.

Garlic Dill Baked Cucumber Chips

(Ready in about 3hour 15 mins:| Serving 16 | Difficulty: easy)

Per serving: kcal 15, Fat:0.1g, Net carbs:3.7g Protein:0.7g

Ingredients

- Large cucumbers 1

- Dried dill 1 tbsp

- Onion powder 1 tsp

- Garlic powder 1 tsp

- Apple cider vinegar 1 tbsp

- Salt to taste

Instructions

1. Cut the cucumbers thinly into 1/8 "of segments.

2. Place cucumbers on a paper towel in a single layer. Put another paper towel on top and push to pull excess moisture into the cucumber slices. If need be, repeat this step. They're the dryer, the crisper they're going to get when they bake.

3. Placed dry pieces of cucumber in a big mixing bowl.

4. Oven preheated to 200°C.

5. Add the onion powder, garlic powder & apple cider vinegar is mixed in a small mixing bowl. Pour the herbal vinegar mixture over slices of cucumber.

6. Line 2 big cookie sheets with bakery release paper. Place the slices of the cucumber into a single layer on the bakery release paper. Sprinkle with a slight quantity of sea salt.

7. Bake three hrs. or more if needed, half-way through revolving trays.

8. Switch off the heat, then let the trays cool down. It will make them even more crispy.

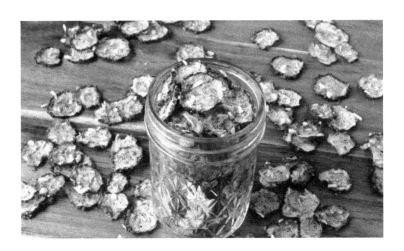

Classic Chocolate Cake Donuts

(Ready in about 33 mins| serving 8 | Difficulty: easy)

Per serving: kcal 123, Fat: 9.2g, net carbs:4.7g, Protein:4.4g

Ingredients

Donuts

- Coconut flour 1/3 cup
- Swerve sweetener 1/3 cup
- Cocoa powder 3 tbsp
- Baking powder 1 tsp
- Salt 1/4 tsp
- Large eggs 4
- Butter melted 1/4 cup
- Vanilla extract 1/2 tsp

- Brewed coffee 6 tbsp

Glaze:

- Powdered Swerve sweetener 1/4 cup

- Cocoa powder 1 tbsp

- Heavy cream 1 tbsp

- Vanilla extract 1/4 tsp

- Water 1 1/2-2 tbsp

Instructions

Donuts:

1. Oven preheated to 325f, & grease well the donut plate.

2. Whisk your coconut powder/flour, the sweetener, cocoa powder, baking soda & salt together in the medium dish. Add the potatoes, butter warmed, & vanilla extract, & mix in the water just until mixed.

3. Split the flour into donut pan pools. If you've got a 6-well donut the tray, you'll need to put in plenty.

4. Bake for 16-20 mins, until donuts are tucked and solid. Remove and allow it to cool in the saucepan for 10 mins, then turn it onto a cooling rack to cool

Glaze:

1. Mix all together concentrated sweetener & powder of cocoa into a shallow med cup. Apply the strong vanilla & cream, then whisks it to blend.

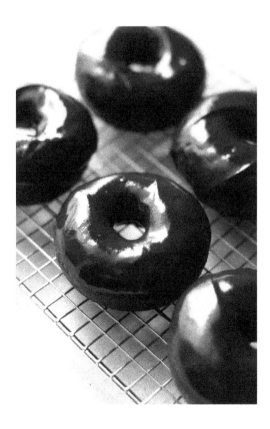

Chocolate Brownie Energy Bites

(Ready in about 30 mins| serving 24 | Difficulty: easy)

Per serving: kcal 179, fat: 16.47g, net carbs:6.56g, Protein:4.29g

Ingredients

Energy bites:

- Coconut oil or butter 1/2 cup
- Unsweetened cocoa powder 1/3 cup
- Swerve sweetener 1/3 cup
- Lightly beaten egg 1
- Almond flour Honeyville 1 cup
- Coconut shredded 1 cup
- Protein powder unflavored 1/2 cup
- Chopped walnuts 1/3 cup

- Coconut flour 2 tbsp

Instructions

Energy Bites:

2. Line the cookie Sheet with bakery release paper

3. Put the butter oil in the med saucepan on med heat. Add the chocolate powder and the sweetener, then stir in the egg and simmer for 5 min. Now remove it from heat.

4. Stir together all the almond meal, chopped coconut, protein powder, diced nuts & coconut Flour in a medium dish. Mix it into saucepan until it's well combined.

5. Shape roll mixture onto balls with the hands using the tablespoon, then lay on the prepared cookie sheet. There are around 24 balls that Will be having. Set a cookie sheet in the refrigerator.

Coating Of chocolate:

1. Place the little metal/ceramic bowl over a cup of slowly boiling water, ensuring the bowl's bottom does not enter the bath.

2. Melt together chocolate & butter when mol ten.

3. Drop bites of icy energy into the Chocolate 1 at the moment, then covers well. To extract extra Cocoa, choose a fork to take it out And softly touch a fork on the surface of the tub. Put back onto the cookie sheet, Lined with waxed sheets. Let's Set.

Chocolate Coconut Candies

(Ready in about 20 mins| serving 24 | Difficulty: easy)

Per serving: kcal 240, Fat: 25g, Net carbs:5g, Protein:2g

Ingredients

Coconut candies:

- Coconut butter 1/2 cup

- Kelapo coconut oil 1/2 cup

- Shredded coconut unsweetened 1/2 cup

- Powdered Swerve sweetener 3 tbsp

Chocolate topping:

- Cocoa butter 1 & 1/2 ounces
- Unsweetened chocolate 1 ounce
- Powdered Swerve sweetener 1/4 cup
- Cocoa powder 1/4 cup
- Vanilla extract 1/4 tsp

Instructions

1. For sweets, line up a tiny-muffin Tray with twenty small paper liners.
2. In a shallow saucepan, mix the coconut Fat & coconut oil on low heat. Remove to melted & clean, then Apply crushed coconut & sweetener when mixed.
3. Divide the mixture into ready tiny muffin cups & freeze for around 30 minutes, until solid.
4. Mix cocoa butter & unflavored chocolate in a bowl placed Over just a pan of boiling water for chocolate coating. Mix until It melts.

5. Mix in sifted powdered sugar after which mix Cocoa powder until its smooth
6. Stir in the vanilla extract & remove it from heat.
7. Chocolate spoon coating over cool coconut Sweets and having it cool, around fifteen minutes.
8. If you are using pre-packed chocolate, then only melt & spoon over the cold coconut filling.
9. Sweets could be kept over A week at the kitchen countertop.

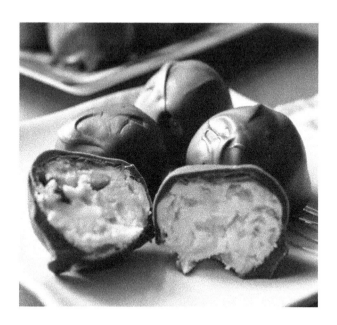

THANK YOU

Thank you for choosing *Ketogenic Diet: Snacks Cookbook* for improving your cooking skills! I hope you enjoyed the recipes while making them and tasting them! If you're interested in learning new recipes and new meals to cook, go and check out the other books of the serie.